RESILIENCE

by Elliot Berger

(Bipolar Depression and the Hand I was Dealt)

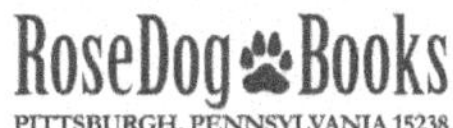

RoseDog Books
PITTSBURGH, PENNSYLVANIA 15238

RoseDog Books
585 Alpha Drive, Suite 103
Pittsburgh, PA 15238
Visit our website at *www.rosedogbookstore.com*

ISBN: 979-8-89211-322-9
eISBN: 979-8-89211-820-0

Dedicated to my parents,
Herman and Pearl Berger.

ACKNOWLEDGMENTS

With much love I want to publicly thank my daughters, Abigail and Amanda, for their love and support during the rough times and through my recovery.

Special gratitude goes to my sister Jackie, who has always had my back and urged me to start exercising and much more—essentially planting the seeds of my recovery— and still encourages me to be my best self every day.

And I am indebted to Pastor Ralphael Jefferson of Jefferson Temple in Bellport, New York, and his wife, Laurie, Direct Lady of the parish, for their friendship and much more.

A special thanks to my cousin Gary for his invaluable assistance.

A thank you to the Management of the Agency for giving me the opportunity to work in a Helping Profession with individuals with special needs. Also a thank you to management and the entire staff for making the job an enjoyable one. This has been a dream of mine for quite some time.

A thank you to Mary for her fine editing work.

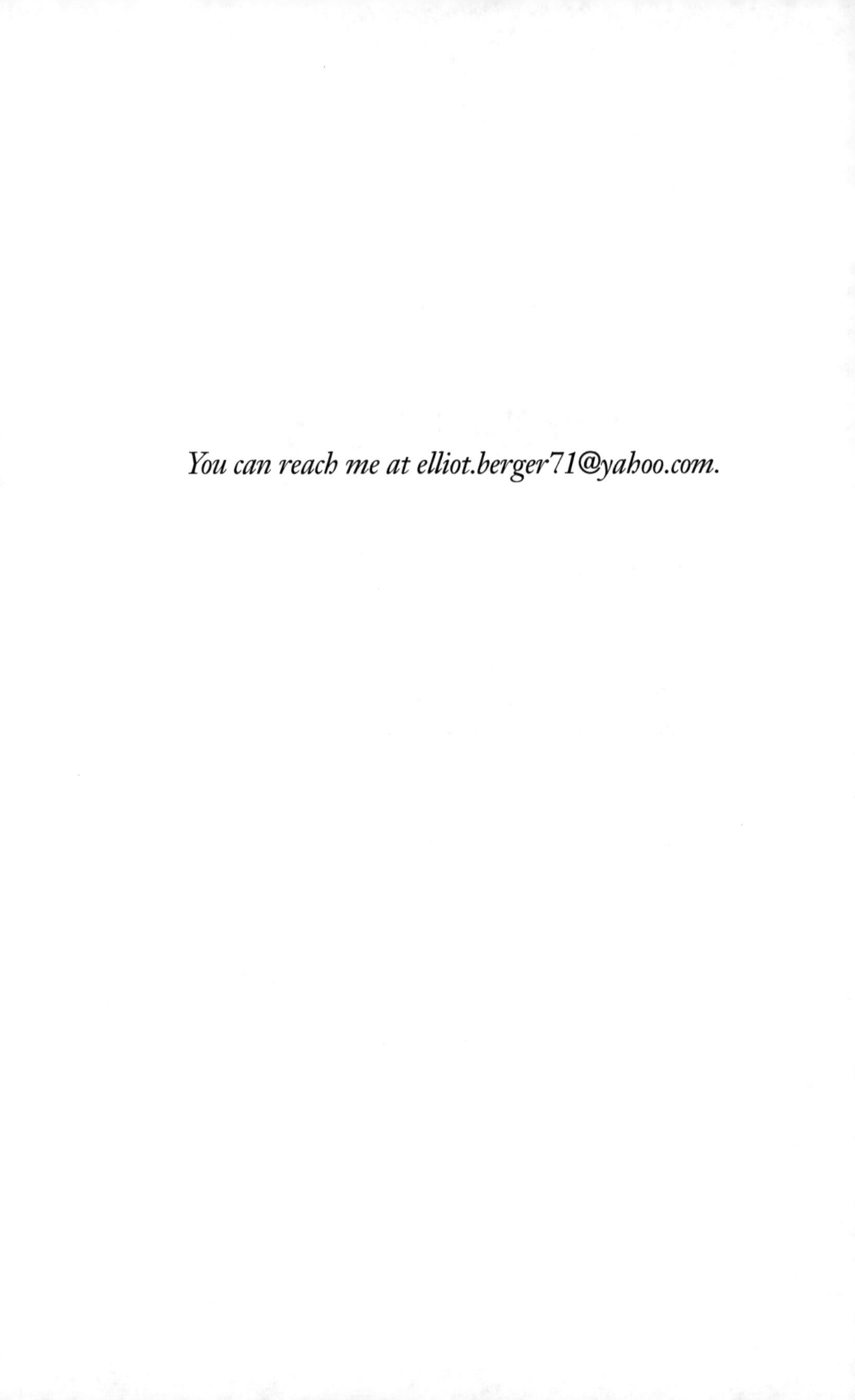

You can reach me at elliot.berger71@yahoo.com.

TABLE OF CONTENTS

INTRODUCTION

It was a cold winter Sunday morning. I found myself in an unfamiliar neighborhood at the Pentecostal church owned by Reverend Jefferson. Little did I know before the service, I would find myself on the dias telling my story. The event would change my life.

I was behind the register at the local Pharmacy in Amityville, New York, where I worked part-time, in the winter of 2021. Reverend Ralphael Jefferson came into the store with his wife, Laurie; I had met the Jeffersons on their previous visits and we were getting to know each other over time. We almost always spent a few minutes chatting about what was going on in our lives. On that day, I started talking about my illness that was diagnosed as bipolar depression, what I had been going through because of it—the struggles and the triumph. The pastor and Lorraine were curious about my story. I might have thought I was over-sharing at the time, or perhaps even complaining, but they were genuinely interested in the challenges I had come up against, especially regarding my disorder, and how I had handled them.

Reverend Jefferson invited me to attend his church as his guest, even though I am Jewish, and I was happy to accept. That Sunday, during the service—and without any kind of warning—he called me up to the pulpit and asked me to share the story of how I had climbed out of my depression. Reverend Jefferson explained his request in simple words: He thought I had something to say.

I was a little taken aback, but I walked to the front of the church and started telling my story to the congregation. As I talked, within five minutes I realized the pastor was right—I do have something to say. It's a message that can be useful to anyone who has suffered with depression. I had an illness that can be treated with great success.

There is no stigma attached to it, any more than if you had been diagnosed with diabetes, or arthritis, or a sinus infection. One thing I've learned along the way, and one message I hope to convey in this book, is that no one did anything to bring this on. There is no culpability, the illness is no one's fault. Some of the most famous celebrities have been depressed, including Lady Gaga, Bruce Springsteen, Olympic swimming champion Michael Phelps, and former First Lady Michelle Obama. All of them have been treated successfully for their illness. Winston Churchill, Ernest Hemingway, Vincent Van Gogh, Ludwig von Beethoven, and countless other historical figures likewise were depressed. Neither fortune nor fame can keep that wolf from the door—only treatment with a capable mental health provider, in my case including therapy, medications and vigorous exercise, can do it.

I was first diagnosed with Bi Polar Depression in January of 1990. I was 38 years old at the time, so I've spent about half of my life with this diagnosed mental illness. There have been rough times, as you will read—some of them *really* rough—but rather than regret, in the long run I realize it was a positive thing for me to have been diagnosed. If I hadn't found a good doctor who pinpointed my illness correctly, I might have gone on and on, spending the rest of my life without being treated. *I had to be diagnosed in order to get treated and turn my life around.*

My motivation for writing this book is the same as my reason for speaking to Rev. Jefferson's congregation: I believe the story of my recovery, and the strategies I've used (backed by scientific research) for climbing out of my own fog, can actually help readers who might be depressed. Doing something to help others has become my motivation in every aspect of my life, in fact—in my career, in my learning, in my family relationships, and in my friendships. You will read about the happiness that comes to me as I work in a "helping profession." Helping others *does* make us feel great—and you'll read some scientific evidence of that, too! It definitely boosts my feelings.

This memoir is divided into three unequal parts:

- **Part 1** – In this first section, you will read about my younger years. I had a great childhood but something happened that would plaque me for much of my adult life.

- **Part 2** – This is a large section of the book, because it encompasses most of my adult life. Here is where I share the kinds of behaviors, moods, and life twists you might expect if you suffer from Bipolar Depression. It was not easy to write about those years, but you deserve the whole story, rough patches and all.

- **Part 3** – This is the most important part of the book. This section documents how I turned my life around and truly started living—and how you can do the same, with control over your life and relationships. In these pages I show readers, in detail, how I began healing, including slip-ups you can avoid if you are alert and honest with yourself, and if you get treatment. You *can* regain your mental health! That is the promise of this book. All of us are a work in progress. This Jewish guy has returned to Rev. Jefferson's Pentecostal church three or four times. Whenever I visit, he still invites me up to the pulpit to share a little more of my story with his parishioners. We have a relationship now. I realize that I still have something to say that might help people, and I'll continue to do so—in front of a congregation, and on these pages. There is a place for all of us, regardless of our age, gender, sexuality, race, or mental health. If we want to live in a world with diversity and inclusivity, it's up to all of us to lead the charge.

PART 1:

MY YOUNGER YEARS

As a young child, I was shy and reserved, almost to a fault. I have memories of my parents trying to jolt me out of my extreme calmness. They weren't being mean, they were just trying to get me to be livelier and more excited about things, and act like a "normal" little boy. (Even saying that sounds like I may have been slightly depressed, doesn't it?) Their tactics rarely worked, though.

Here's an example of my shyness: One day when I was about five years old, my father and I walked into a camera shop. As it turned out, this wasn't a brief stop. I'm guessing we were in there for about an hour—and I stood by his side the entire time and didn't say one word. Even the person helping my dad commented, "Is he always this well-behaved?"

Mostly, though, I think my parents were happy to have such a quiet, easygoing son. "Elliot's a good boy," I heard them say countless times. My aunts would say the same thing; I remember my Aunt Bonnie telling my cousin Jeffrey, "Be like Elliot. He's a good kid." One result of that constant praise was that it created an expectation of me. I had to be the good kid, that already was my reputation, at least as I saw it in my very young eyes. It felt like a kind of pressure on me. As time went on, I was always looking for approval (up to and including my adult years).

Even in the middle of my deep, adult depression, I felt insecure and distrustful, because I wasn't getting approval. People weren't patting me on the head, the way they had when I was younger. And the more I felt that inadequate the more I worried about not getting approval—it was a vicious circle. When I had these thoughts of inadequacy my mood would go flat.

I grew up in Amityville, New York. Most people only know Amityville as the setting for a scary movie (*The Amityville Horror, 1979*), but in reality it is a sweet, picturesque beach village of fewer than 10,000 residents. Located on the southern shore of Long Island, the town is full of well-tended parks and public spaces; Annie Oakley used to visit frequently, and in the early 1900s it was known for the large homes and posh hotels along the bay.

I participated in the kinds of activities that other boys did. I played Little League baseball, rode bicycles and built tree forts. I had mostly a good life growing up. even though I may have had some form of depression as a child. But I didn't realize it until I was grown and looked back. My brother suffered with depression as well, and I'll go into that later. The experts didn't know much about childhood depression back then, but I've included some notes about it at the end of this section.

My mother, Pearl, worked as a bookkeeper; she was born in Brooklyn, New York. My father, Herman, hails from Akron, Ohio. But somehow a large collection of aunts, uncles and cousins landed in and around Amityville, and it was just great to have so many relatives within a 10-minute drive for family gatherings and dinners.

My dad was a modest but successful businessman. Just before I was born, he bought a gas station in Copiague, a Long Island suburb adjacent to Amityville. His garage was the first on the island to offer a free installation when a customer bought a muffler. Some years later, he built an auto parts store next to the station called H & J Auto Parts; I remember stamping catalogs with the name and address of the store when I was about six years old—my first job.

There was also a machine shop in the rear of the store. Dad worked very hard but he also had a little fun with his work, too. One of the funniest examples was his sign on the front door; it read, "Sorry, we are open," and on the reverse side it read, "Hooray, we are closed!"

And he loved to tease the women who came in. He would stand at the counter and shout, "All the women over here," motioning to a spot beside him. Of course, the women would all giggle and obediently walk over to the "women's line." People just loved and respected Dad, and they came from all over the Island to do business with him.

It seemed that he was always around if there was an emergency, and he always did whatever he could to help. I remember one time a fellow had a fishing hook stuck in his finger, with the barb on the end sticking out. People standing nearby tried to pull it out, but couldn't do it. Dad went up to him with his cutting pliers and slowly snipped, snipped, and was very careful. He didn't try to pull it out; Dad knew exactly what he needed to do, and when he had finished cutting out the part of the barb that was sticking out, the rest just came sliding out of the man's finger. There is another story about a man who got his foot stuck in a hole. Two guys were trying to pull his foot out but with no success. Dad saw what was happening and got a can of motor oil and poured it in the hole. The man's foot slid right out. Once again he saved the day.

I continued working in Dad's store through high school and college. I mostly worked at the counter and made deliveries, and Dad sometimes had me driving around to other gas stations and car dealerships to offer our products and services. He was a good, strategic thinker, and he expected more from me than from any of his other workers. Being the boss's son meant absolutely nothing; I had to work hard. He put all the energy he could into his business so he could provide everything we needed, and more besides.

My dad also was an artist. He worked in metal, wood and glass, and he was good at it. Some of his pieces were purely decorative, but many were functional in the house. When he and mom were first married, he made a liquor and china cabinet. They were a set; the liquor cabinet rested on the floor and the china cabinet hung on the wall—and he made these pieces with hand tools (saw, hammer, screw driver and a carving knife), he had no power tools at the time. They were adorned with details and engravings, embellishments and scroll work done with a carving knife that really enhanced their beauty. We still have a roll-top cabinet in our kitchen that Dad made.

I had two siblings, Ronald and Jacqueline. When I wasn't playing baseball with my friends or teammates, we were building tree forts in vacant lots and Ronnie was our "supervisor" who organized us "builders." We would spend hours scavenging vacant lots for wood scraps to use in our creations. We had one friend who was an electrical genius, even as a kid, and he built a phone system from the ground level up to one of our tree forts.

When we played, I still could be that easygoing kid looking for everyone's approval. One example: When I was about five years old, Jackie and her friends used to dress me up in her clothes. My name in those games was "Miss Snodgrass," and I went along with it willingly. In the summer, every day the three of us siblings went to day camp. We would paint, draw, play kickball and put on plays for the other kids. I remember those day camp outings as great fun.

Because our relatives lived nearby, we were able to set in motion the kinds of friendships that sprout early and keep growing. My sister Jackie remembers times when we would go to my cousins' house and I would gather up all their toys and hoard them, not letting any of the other kids play with them. Then I would ride their rocking horse, holding their toys in my arms as if I owned them. Jackie never lets me forget that! I could be a brat when I put my mind to it.

I used to "play doctor" with my female cousins when we were little. You might say I was advanced for my age in that way—we exposed our private parts to each other, though I don't believe we ever touched. My parents kept an empty armoire in their garage, and one of my cousins and I climbed into it one time, closed the doors and exposed ourselves.

That isn't the most serious thing I did as a little kid, though. There was a little girl living upstairs in our home—again, we were about five years old—and she couldn't say my name, Elliot, correctly. She called me "Eddiot," and she used to say, "Eddiot, you marry me."

We had a washing machine at the bottom of the basement stairs, and one day my dad's work clothes were in the washer. We took a couple of our cats and tossed them into the washing machine—and of course, when my father went to retrieve his work clothes, he found the dead cats in there. He instinctively knew who had killed the kitties, and he whipped the living daylights out of me.

I got a lot of earaches when I was a young kid, and once I had an ear infection. Back then, doctors sometimes made house calls, and our family physician, Dr. Gerson, came to our house to check on me. (I was too young to remember much about him, but I remember that he was bald!) He was in our kitchen, sterilizing some hypodermic needles in a frying pan, and when I saw what he was doing, I freaked out. I told my brother to run and get my rubber hatchet, and I proceeded to hit Dr. Gerson over the head with it.

We went into New York City fairly often to visit the museums, the Statue of Liberty, the Empire State Building and other iconic attractions. We often strolled through Chinatown when we were in the City; we would eat at a Chinese restaurant and I remember Dad would always order duck. In winter, we took skiing trips to places like Lake Placid, a resort village in the Adirondacks in northeastern New York State—a onetime site of the Winter Olympics that now hosts winter sports. We also drove to Blair Mountain in the winter. Those ski trips were my favorite family vacations. We traveled to Florida four times I can remember. I could remember on one of those trips to Florida I got lost in the hotel and could not find my way back to Mom and Dad's room. Also on one of the trips we took a ride on a Goodyear Blimp.(Dad sold Goodyear tires and we are able to ride for free). In the summer, we sometimes went to Lake George, an upscale vacation town and lake in the Adirondacks. These vacations and outings weren't cheap, especially the trips to Florida,(a couple of times we drove and we also took a plane the other times) but Mom and Dad somehow managed to pay for them. They wanted us to experience different things, different places.

Then there were the frequent family parties at our house, and at the homes of our cousins. Life was good—usually. At times I think maybe there was too much going on for me to feel depressed in those years, though my overly shy, quiet behavior does tell another story.

In high school, I discovered music in a big way—so much so that even now, I think it would have been nice to have been an accomplished musician. One of my fondest memories of my mother, who died a few years ago, was when she, Ronnie and I went to a rock concert in Central Park. The Animals were the featured performers Led by Eric Burdon, they were part of the "British Invasion" of the 1960s, famous for such songs as "House of the Rising Sun" and "Don't Let Me Be Misunderstood." My mom sat there the whole time, never complaining. She was a cool mom, she really was.

In her later years, Mom was diagnosed with Parkinson's disease. This did not stop her from enjoying life. Mom went with Jackie and I to a concert in the city. The featured performer was a group called "Rocktopia". They were a five-piece rock band and a 30-member symphony orchestra fusing classical music with classic rock. Also, there was the time when Mom and Jackie and myself went to a country music festival that lasted for five hours; she sat outside in her wheelchair the entire time and listened to the music. Mom wasn't there just for the music. This was also a social event for her. She made friends with the people around her. It was just a wonderful day for her. This made me happy.

My parents were always hip, and not only musically. The Beatles were hot when I was a teenager, and my father actually took time to listen to their music, pull it apart a little bit, to understand what they were trying to do. He even got into discussions with me and my friends about Beatles songs. Dad would say they were "way out," and my friends called him a "cool guy" because their parents thought the Beatles were just long hair freaks . He thought that Bob Dylan was a poet who was ahead of his time. These were good examples of the differences between my parents and others in our circle. I am so proud of my parents.

Around this time, I played rhythm guitar in a rock band with three friends—a bass player, a lead guitarist and a drummer. We named ourselves "An Act of Love and Kindness." We all sang, and we weren't bad. My brother Ronnie and myself rode our bikes about 20 miles to buy an electric guitar so we could play it in our band.

One day in 1968 I was about 16. The four of us decided to organize a "battle of the bands" with two other bands. One of the other bands sounded better than us, and we were glad they decided to play in the "battle" because we knew they would attract a bigger crowd.

We rented the local roller rink, put up flyers across town—even in the places where the "tough guys" hung out—and charged admission, though we didn't share that money with the other two bands. We all played to a full house; the roller rink was packed, and after paying rent for the rink (plus a fee for a sink that somehow got broken), each member of our band took home forty dollars.

Another memorable high school adventure was my trip to Europe. I was taking a class in French, and the teacher mentioned a private school in Manhattan that was sponsoring a trip, taking kids from all over the country on a tour of Europe. I told my mom and dad that I wanted to go, and being the kind of parents they were—the kind who wanted their kids to see and experience other places and cultures—they were all for it.

I worked to help pay for part of the trip, but my parents paid for most of it. Again, that was the kind of behavior that set them apart from other parents I knew. It was a seven-week junket, and I was the only student from my school who went. I saw Brussels, Rome, Geneva and, of course, Paris. Looking back, Rome and Paris were my favorite cities. I remember one guy selling jewelry on a street corner in Paris, and I tried to communicate with him using my high-school French. I was thinking this was great that I could communicate with him. At the end of the conversation he says to me in English "by the way what part of Brooklyn are you from". Well that really burst my bubble. He not only new I was from the states but detected a Brooklyn accent. We had a good laugh about that. He was an American and he probably missed America a little bit. I bought a couple of trinkets from him for my mom and sister.

Other than playing in the band and taking that big trip to Europe, though, I was very apathetic in high school. I didn't play sports or join any clubs; I would go to school and then come right home or go to my job. The band was my only activity beyond work and school. Aside from a couple of friends I made in my freshman year of college, I wasn't at all interested in organized school activities, or in socializing in general. It might have been a symptom of my developing depression. My grades were fine; I maintained a "B" average.

But high school also marked the beginning of feeling odd. I wasn't a perfectly behaved teenager, though I didn't get into real trouble, and I only smoked cigarettes for a month or two. I didn't enjoy smoking—suddenly I couldn't walk up a flight of stairs without being out of breath, and for me that was a terrible feeling. I figured smoking wasn't worth it.

I did a fair amount of drugs, though—I smoked pot; this was back when kids did a lot of weed. And I used hashish and some acid. Now I wonder if my drugs might have been partly responsible for my depression.

I can remember the day when I knew something inside my brain was different. I was still in high school then, walking down a hall by myself, when something went off in my head. It's hard to describe in words, but it was like a shift in my awareness. I felt that I had actually shifted between dimensions, if that makes sense. Something felt almost broken. Years later, my psychiatrist and I talked about it, and we speculated that I may have been living with low-grade depression for the better part of my life; this "shift" was that part of me, the part that was ill, coming to the surface. From then on, I was more aware of my feelings than I had been before.

PART 2:

THIS IS WHAT DEPRESSION LOOKS LIKE

Passover is a heartwarming holiday ritual for Jewish families. It is our major spring holiday, a true celebration when we come together and commemorate the liberation of Israelites from Egyptian slavery and the sparing of their first-born children. The holiday lasts for seven days, marked by holy meals and special prayer services; during these days we are reminded of how precious freedom is, and how, when things go wrong, we can pick ourselves up and start over.

One of the highlights of Passover, is the Seder dinner, and one Monday in 1985 we were at my Uncle Louis's and Aunt Evelyn's home for the Seder. It was a fairly big family event, with maybe 15 people present. I was with my wife, Margaret, my beautiful daughters, Abigail and Amanda, and my cousins had come with their children. My parents were there, along with my sister Jackie and my brother Ronnie. It was a fun, meaningful holiday; first we read from the Haggadah, the book that tells the story of the Jews' bondage in Egypt and how Moses helped them to break free. Each person gets a chance to read a part of the story. After the reading was over the dinner became a social event and there was plenty to eat, chicken soup with matzo balls. The main course was turkey and brisket, along with sweet potatoes and stuffing, with spinach and asparagus on the side.

When it was time for dessert, Aunt Evelyn really showed off her baking skills. That night she had made Mandel (almond) bread and Rugelach. After dessert, it was time for the youngest kids to look for the "Hidden Matza"

We said our good-byes at about 7:00 p.m. We were home by about 8:30, said good-night to the girls and had them in bed by 9:00. Then the phone rang, and my world fell apart.

We lived in New Jersey in a very upscale community, and I had a great job that paid well. I worked at a firm that was a key player in the New Jersey bond market. I was an Underwriter; I assisted municipalities in raising money in the bond market. I put together a syndicate of Wall Street dealers and managed the dealers in bidding on municipal bond issues around the country. It was my responsibility to develop consensus as to the pricing of the bond issues amongst these dealers in the group I managed. The group that offers the lowest net interest cost (NIC) to the issuer of the bonds wins the deal.

Every small, subtle shift in the bidding matters. One group could bid a 6.74 net interest cost, while one of their competitors could bid a 6.75 NIC, and those who bid 6.74 would get the deal. There might be many groups bidding on any issue, and we often would compete with large banks, large corporations in the financial services industry and smaller firms as well. Multi-million-dollar projects were at stake—they might be for water and sewer plants, erecting a school building, and similar undertakings. On larger deals we would be one of many dealers in a syndicate. It was my job to decide whether or not to stay in the deal and commit the firm's capital.

When we were the winning bidder, it was exciting, and I had a certain cachet. Buying the deal, and coming out on top, was only half of the process. Once we achieved that, we needed to sell the bonds—a critical step because if we couldn't sell all the bonds, we could lose money.

The company I worked for got involved with repos. If you remember, this was a national story. The way it worked was, that my company would borrow money from banks on a short-term basis, and while they held the banks' funds, they paid interest on those loans. The problem was, the owners of my company were using the borrowed money for their own personal use—a private jet, expensive cars, and a French chef in the company lunch room.

When another trading firm wasn't able to meet their repo obligations, the news spread and the customers of our company, got nervous and called for their money. That started the downward spiral, and some, if not all of it, was missing.

Needless to say, we went out of business. The call I received that evening, after the Seder dinner, was from a co-worker. He had phoned to tell me the company was finished and I was out of a job.

It was a shame, really, because our municipal trading and underwriting activities were first-class and well-respected in the industry. Some of the salesmen had parked a portion of their wages with the firm as deferred compensation. They lost their money.

The problem for me was, I was out of work and had to support my family. Even though I lived in an affluent neighborhood and had been earning a great salary, I had very little money in the bank.

I had no choice but to sign up for unemployment, but that didn't bring in enough money to make ends meet. I needed more. A friend of mine helped me find a job working for a construction company; most of the time, that job had me cleaning up construction sites, including disposing of discarded pieces of wood into massive garbage hoppers. I was grateful for the income but the work was hardly satisfying, and I only stayed in that job for a short time.

As much as I adore my daughters, starting a family when we did was unrealistic. There had been no thoughts about whether I was ready, career-wise or financially, or whether we would be able to survive on one income. But Margaret was ready emotionally and physically. I was dealing with emotions, not reality, but I went along in my easygoing way, as I had done since I was a little boy, always doing whatever it took to get approval. What I failed to realize was, *if I was not happy with myself, how in the world can I make someone else happy?* Margaret and I met in 1975 a year after I got out of college. We got married in 1976. Abigail was born in 1977 and Amanda came later in 1980.

Still, I had been excited when Abigail and Amanda were born, though those wonderful events didn't transform me into a happy person. I couldn't handle the responsibility, I didn't know how to be happy, and that prevented me from being an involved, dedicated father and husband.

I was always looking to do something different with my career. I started thinking I wanted to start my own business. I would go into bookstores looking for self-help books on how to start a business. Every time I walked past a bookstore, I would go in and sometimes come out with a new book on starting a business. Other times, I would buy a more general self-improvement book. That went on for years; the feeling would consume me. I wasn't going to start a business at that time, it was just a persistent wish because I was so unhappy. I was always wishing for a different life—even when I went to the beach I would watch the birds, standing there and wishing I was a bird because I was not happy in the life I had.

At the same time, true depression set in. I would look at other families—they seemed to be so happy. I wished I could be like them. I was sad then, and it makes me sad today that I couldn't completely enjoy my family during those years.

More symptoms: I was also losing my ability to function well. My attention span wasn't good. I couldn't even hear what people were saying. A fog was setting in.

I always felt as if I were under pressure, and often that pressure was about getting someone's approval. Since I was a small child, as I've mentioned, I had been looking for approval. In the middle of my depression I was very desperate that I didn't feel that I was getting the approval I needed. It was a vicious circle—the more desperate I got, the more I worried about not getting approval. It made me feel alone in the world (and depressed).

I could not find work in New York. So I placed a position wanted ad in a Financial Services industry publication. I got a response from a company in Ohio. I went out there to interview and take a look at the area. They made me an offer which I accepted and started in January 1986. I was to promote the purchase and sale of municipal bonds. I had an assistant who worked with me. The firm I worked for was an investment firm with approximately 120 brokers and about 40 support staff. There were 5 branch offices. The company rented an apartment for me. Margaret and the girls came that April. Before they relocated to Ohio, I would fly home every other weekend. On the weekends when I stayed in Ohio, I sometimes hung out with people from work, going to restaurants and bars, drinking together, visiting with their families and children, and generally having a good time. Having a good time would get out of hand when I went out with a group of people from work. We went to a restaurant where there was music. We were all having a good time. There was a woman in the group that attached herself to me. She was very pretty. She asked me to dance with her and I enjoyed that. When the music got slow she led me out on the dance floor. We got close and I was getting a bit turned on. This group and I would go out a few times. One night this woman asked me to drive her home. We got to her home and she asked me if I wanted to come in. I agreed. We went upstairs to her apartment. We sat on her couch and talked. This was about 10:30 p.m. She was very attractive and I was feeling good to be in her company alone. At one point I asked if I could kiss her. She obliged and we started to kiss simply and then we got very passionate and we laid close to each other on the couch. I was turned on and I knew I could have sex with her if I wanted. I resisted. We grinded against each other and kissed deeply. This went on all night. I kept resisting the desire to have sex. Then at about 4:00 a.m. my will was weak and I gave in. Her body was beautiful. I left her house at about 5 a.m. I felt that there was a fundamental change in me for the worst. I was now a cheat. Some people could have an affair and it would not bother them. This bothered me. I was not made to be a cheat. This feeling, this act would help contribute to my deep depression. But I was missing my own family and children. My boss was a relatively young guy and we liked each other. I must say that my boss and my friends there were very good to me. They made me feel at home.

Margaret had issues that made our marriage challenging. She at times made me choose between her and my family. We had been married for 11 years by the time we all moved to Ohio; our daughters Abigail and Amanda were 10 and seven. I really tried to be a good father, but I don't think I was able to give them the attention they needed all the time. I was nearly all consumed with my job and career, and the depression stopped me from growing as a person or giving my mental health the care and attention it needed.

It would be hard to over-state the grip that depression had on me. I was on the cusp of entering a chapter of my life where the way I handled my job would nearly destroy me. Being depressed was like having a perpetual cloud over me, regardless of any positive things that happened to me. As the depression became stronger, the cloud would get thicker and was progressively difficult for me to function. Paranoia was a constant symptom; even when I now had a job in Ohio, I was afraid of the FBI and the SEC (Securities and Exchange Commission), even though I never committed a crime or did anything those agencies would want to investigate.

I became involved in an important project. We were going to assist a local municipality that needed to raise money. Over the following year, that project would consume virtually all of my mental energy. I had hardly any physical or emotional energy left for Margaret and the girls. The stress was palpable and constant, and deepened my depression.

Not that Margaret would have been happy anyway. When Margaret and the girls drove into the town that April, Margaret's heart sank. But for Margaret, the city represented nothing good. It was a depressing place, with boarded-up windows on businesses, abandoned houses and decaying steel mills. It closely resembled Buffalo, where she had spent a most unhappy childhood. It was a constant reminder of deep unhappiness she wanted to leave behind. Every day, she thought she was looking at Buffalo again.

So, moving to the city was a challenge for Margaret on a few levels. Getting used to living in a new city is never easy, and the time I spent on my project at work, which would turn out to be very successful, would contribute greatly to our deteriorating relationship. We settled in a small town in every sense. Work and play became intertwined. I joined the Rotary Club which took me further away from my family and cut the time I would have been spending with them. I screwed up. I should have provided time for my family, but I truly didn't have it in me to be an attentive father. I was over-involved in my own activities, which took a toll on our marriage.

We had rented an apartment for four months while we had our house built. During those months, we lived among countless unopened boxes, but it would have been worth it, had we been otherwise happy: the new house was a beautiful center-hall colonial, with four bedrooms and two and a half baths. The kitchen counters were tiled in a vibrant blue to contrast with the white cabinets, and any floors that weren't carpeted were outfitted in pickled pine. We put a family room off the kitchen, complete with a fireplace and large glass doors leading to the backyard. The primary bedroom had a large *en suite* bath with a Jacuzzi tub. It was a house that we never would have been able to afford in New York.

I thought that building a snazzy new home would lift Margaret's spirits, but we moved into it in August and by February she was ready to sell the house and move. She was lonely, though I wasn't really aware of her loneliness in the moment—I was too focused on work and the Rotary Club to pay much attention to Margaret and the girls. My boss wanted me to be comfortable, though he hadn't seen Margaret's unhappiness.

Meanwhile Margaret wanted to sell the house and move (we were in the house for only six months). We put a "For Sale" sign on the property. News travels fast in a small town, and the next day my boss questioned me about selling the house. Margaret and I had conjured up a story; she was going to work for her brother, an attorney in Cleveland. I wasn't comfortable about lying to anyone, let alone someone I liked and respected, so making up this story was a major source of stress for me.

I was going to move to Cleveland with Margaret and the girls, and I told my boss I would be able to commute. It was a one-hour commute, but we hadn't found a new home in Cleveland. Margaret wanted to move back to New York, so we drove back there one weekend. I was going through the motions, pretending to go along with her idea, though I secretly wanted to keep my job. And to add to the stress, we had to vacate our house that we'd sold, and we had nowhere to go; for all practical purposes, we were homeless. We ended up staying at a motel for a few nights.

It felt like forever that we didn't have a home because it was so stressful, not knowing where we would land, but we found an apartment quickly. We were able to rent it on a month-to-month basis. Eventually we bought a house in Cleveland, and I began my one-hour (each way) daily commute.

But the fact was, my job performance was slipping. In my job, I had to make decisions all the time; some were simple and many were extremely complex. One of the transactions I could execute was to fill an order for a municipal bond. I could simply buy a bond from another dealer. The other thing I could do is bid on a bond through a broker. This requires a special skill. But I got to the point where I wasn't making decisions and my focus was very limited. It was like I was in a fog all the time—paranoia, my constant companion, was more of a burden than ever.

I thought the world was against me, and I still worried that the SEC and FBI were after me. It's strange that I could believe this without questioning it. That was Paranoia. I also thought the feds were watching me from helicopters. Maybe, I thought, the people I worked with were spying on me. I knew they were observing me, and seeing that I wasn't performing well. It was as if I had a bag over my head; my ears were not hearing everything and I wasn't processing all of the information presented to me.

It is challenging to describe what depression feels like. In the worst times, I felt hopeless and lonely. I was tired and had brain fog. I describe brain fog as not being able to concentrate and I had difficulty processing what people were saying to me.

I wasn't sleeping well and the paranoia never left.

As an aside, I thought it was paranoia that stayed with me for many years, even as I was recovering.

The company wanted to float a bond issue for a water and sewer treatment plant in 1987. I was working on the project with another broker/dealer in Ohio. Because my judgement wasn't working, I completely missed the mark on the pricing of the issue. Those numbers are a bit subjective and depend on a number of factors—but it was my job to weigh all of those factors and pinpoint the best pricing. I failed to do that. The firm we partnered with developed a pricing that was more realistic and worked for the issuer and our two firms. I was happy with the way things turned out.

Finally, while Margaret and I were living in Cleveland, she and I separated. I got an apartment, and started socializing with my co-workers again. I hung out with a few friends from the office and would spend a little time with their families—I was having a good time! What I didn't realize was that I was in a manic phase. I was high-energy, felt invincible, and didn't need much sleep—or so I thought. And when I took a moment to reflect, I knew that I was lonely for Margaret and the girls. This manic phase lasted for about one year. On more than one occasion I asked Margaret if she would take me back. She refused. She became very worried about me and called my family to express her concern.

After Margaret and I separated, I would visit my daughters. During one of those visits, Margaret and I got into a major heated argument, and something in me snapped. For the first time, I really voiced my opinion in a strong way. One of my lifelong issues was letting people have too much control over me, and not standing up for myself—probably because I was still that little boy, looking for approval. But this time I *did* stand up for myself, and I think we were both surprised. After that, both Margaret and I felt better about each other, and we became friends.

We filed for divorce in 1989. When we had our last meeting with our attorneys, Margaret and I sat outside the room, talking as if we'd been friends our entire lives. We remained friendly until she died in 2020.

After a while, I started to date again, but it would be 10 years before I would remarry. I did meet one beautiful, blonde, sexy woman who had two children. I thought our relationship would go somewhere, and I invited her to come to New York to meet my family. That meeting never happened, and I was starting to lose my energy—the manic phase was winding down. I no longer felt invincible. My "need" for not much sleep morphed into an inability to sleep, and I was now entering a deep depression. I drove to work one morning as usual, found a spot in the parking garage—and never got out of the car. I sat there, and sat…the entire day, from 8:00 in the morning until the work day ended at 5:00. I don't remember how my boss knew I had spent the day sitting in my car, but it was one of the very lowest points in my depression history. My boss gave me the name of a psychiatrist who might help me. I did make an appointment with the psychiatrist, who prescribed Prozac, a popular drug that's prescribed for depression, obsessive-compulsive disorder and anxiety disorders. It boosts the serotonin levels in the brain and is supposed to have a positive effect on the patient's mood, emotions and sleep. But the Prozac didn't help me at all, and my mental health continued to deteriorate. The worst symptoms of the depression lasted about one year.

I was in a fog, I wasn't functioning, and everyone was aware of my condition; it was obvious just from observing my behavior. Jackie was in touch with a couple of my friends and tried to persuade me to come home to Amityville, but I resisted. Finally, on December 1, 1989 I was fired. The company felt I wasn't functioning. The next day, after four years in Ohio, a friend drove me to the airport and I was home in Amityville that night.

Back on Long Island, I was with my mother and sister in a psychiatrist's office the next day. He admitted me to the hospital immediately. (Over the years, I've been hospitalized three times.) I was placed in a ward with other patients who suffered from all sorts of mental conditions, so I was uncomfortable there. The hospital ward I was in was very austere. There were three to four people in each bed oom. There were approximately 30 patients. We were up every morning at 7:00 a.m. We got our meds and then went to the common area for breakfast. There was a kitchen/large livingroom with couches and TV. We were responsible for keeping our bedroom and common area neat and did our laundry once a week. There was a washer and dryer on the ward. My doctor would visit me every day to see how I was feeling. Also, one of the staff would meet with me, daily to see how I was doing. The doctors wrestled with two issues: the first was to find a medication that was effective, that I could tolerate. One antidepressant called Pamelor had me trying to swallow my tongue, which was incredibly scary.

The other issue was deciding whether to treat my depression with shock therapy. Electroconvulsive therapy (ECT), sometimes called "electroshock therapy," sends an electric current through the brain, causing a surge of electrical activity in the brain—in effect, a seizure. The aim is to relieve symptoms of certain mental health problems. Electroshock therapy actually causes changes in the patient's brain chemistry, quickly reversing the symptoms. It's administered to about 100,000 people a year in psychiatric hospitals or psych units. One of the mental conditions it's used for is severe depression.

The doctors decided to go ahead with ECT. I was sedated and electrodes were attached to my head. When I awoke, my head was surprisingly clear. Sometimes it causes temporary side effects, such as headaches, confusion, or a memory loss, according to the American Psychiatric Association, but I was given three shock therapy treatments over time and suffered zero side effects. It helped me for about two months.

After spending about three weeks in the hospital in the program I was taken to my parents' home—the place where I would feel most safe. I was told to schedule a visit with the doctor every two weeks. The doctor put me on Lithium which he eventually took me off. My parents, along with my sister Jackie—my strongest "support group"—flew to Pittsburgh, drove the rest of the way to my apartment and packed everything up. They even drove my car back to New York. Around that time, the doctor met with me and my family to educate us about the effects of my mental condition, which he diagnosed as bipolar disorder. (I had just come off a two-year cycle, so the bipolar diagnosis was correct at that time. In more recent years, my illness evolved and I was depressed but no longer bipolar.) My family was worried about me and my father was particularly distraught about my condition.

I was now unemployed, but I don't believe I could have handled a job at that time. Still, it meant I had a lot of time on my hands. I spent much of that time bonding with my father; the two of us built a small building in the back-yard—sort of an oversized shed, 20 feet by 12 feet. We did all of the work our-selves, except for pouring the concrete slab. Dad wanted me to be active so he felt that this project would be a good way to keep busy.

One of my cousins approached me to come and work with him in his plumbing supply business. I appreciated his offer, but I declined because I had decided that what I really wanted was to run my own business.

During the next three years, I tried to start an import/export business. I wanted to deal in electronics. My father encouraged me—"if you don't do it now, when will you do it?" He said. Of course, I had no experience in imports and exports and knew nothing about that field. I spent $7,000 of my own money "preparing" for my new business, getting business cards made, having brochures designed, producing catalogs. I even set up my own phone line and fax line and a dedicated room in my parents' home. I had all the infrastructure that any business needs, but I had no customers.

Everything I did cost a lot of money, including overseas calls and mailings. I ended up needing financial support from my parents, and over those three years they gave me approximately $75,000. My daughter Amanda told me I should go out and get a regular job! I was then dating a really nice woman for two years; she waited all that time for me to establish my business and get it running.

But it was a complete failure. I spent three years chasing large transactions, but in the end, I had to give up the idea. I did have one buyer in Queens and made samples for him. This buyer was a very large manufacturer of electrical wiring devices (ie switches, outlets, surge protectors etc) The device is a very simple porcelain lamp holder. They are typically used in basements or attics. He gave us an order for a container load, 4,000 pieces. But this delivery was coming from China. The quality was good, the price was right but they couldn't deliver the product on time. I was working with an agent on Long Island.

Following my business failure, I was able to get a job telemarketing for a window manufacturer and then telemarketing for an alarm system manufacturer. Telemarketing was definitely not a very satisfying line of work, but I didn't care because it wasn't going to be a career. What's more I actually was very good at it. The alarm company I worked for went out of business. I could not find any other work in telemarketing. Then I went to work for Target for about a year, stocking shelves and helping customers.

Somehow, it occurred to me that being a home health aide would be more satisfying. I did that for more than a year and made a decision that this is still my personal commitment: I want to be in a helping profession. I'm not sure when that notion occurred to me, but I still am pursuing it. I never stopped wanting to earn a living by helping people, and I'll share more about that particular ambition—and what I did about it—later in the book.

As a home health aide, I worked part-time helping patients with whatever tasks they couldn't handle themselves. Sometimes I ran errands, or made their lunch, or helped them shower. They weren't terribly ill, but most were older and couldn't drive. They just needed some help. It was somewhat rewarding and helped me solidify my ambition to help people. I took a course at BOCES (Boards of Cooperative Educational Services) to become a medical assistant but couldn't find a job in that field. The work wasn't there. I still needed to make a decent living. I did not want just another telemarketing job.

One day in 1996, I noticed an ad from a small company in the financial services sector. This was my background. I had been a stock broker and a bond underwriter and trader but I no longer had a license. I was drowning with no direction. Little did I know that when I made the call to this company, it would mark the start of a long journey to turn my life around and find success again. Along the way, I was given opportunities that I seized. I managed to climb out of a hole of depression and failure. So I joined the company as a telemarketer, a skill at which I excelled. My job was to persuade stockbrokers to move themselves and their book of business to the company I worked for. I did well, and soon was transferred to the operations department, where transactions were executed. The company sponsored me to get my securities license (series 7). My original license lapsed because I was not in the business. This is a significant development because now, with the license I can go anywhere.

It had been about four years since I'd had a "normal" job. Some of the work was tedious and some was working with independent brokers, individuals who were self-employed contractors with their own offices. Those independent reps took an 80 to 85 percent cut of the commission, and the company took the remaining 15 to 20 percent of the commission. The commissions were from the sale of mutual funds, stocks and bonds and insurance products. In just two short months, I was promoted to Operations Manager. Life was good. I moved into an apartment, the second story of a Cape Cod style home.

This small company employed just 15 people and supported about 100 independent brokers. It was all manageable for someone like me, just getting back into full-time work, and I felt comfortable there. I personally managed a staff of seven individuals.

Shortly thereafter, the business was sold to a veterinarian from England who didn't know the first thing about the financial services industry. He was an older man. The president and another man, took me to dinner one night and offered me a lucrative position. They said they would pay me $65,000 with a guaranteed $20,000 bonus, but I told them I wasn't interested. The business was soon liquidated, and once more, I was out of work.

Thankfully, another company sought me out. They wanted to hire some of the brokers, who were the producers. They also were looking for some support staff, and one of the brokers recommended me to the owner of this company.

The principals made me an attractive offer. My job was to transition the brokers book of business to this company. Also, I wore another hat when I assisted in building the company website. Later this company, would become a subsidiary of a major insurance company. I would be there until 2008.

One day, in 1994 I was riding the subway in New York City, and a homeless man was selling a newspaper. I took a closer look and saw an article about dating. The article recommended a caption for a singles ad in a magazine or newspaper, so I bought the paper and used the caption I had seen: "Looking for a partner, not a date." I received an astonishing 120 responses from the ad! Out of those, I actually met about 20 women, and finally met Judy, the woman who would become my second wife. Judy and I dated for 5 years before we got engaged and we were married in 1999.

What really created a lot of stress for me, and eventually serious depression, was being around Judy's kids while they grew up. They would move back and forth between Judy's house and her Ex's home. Every time there was a move Judy and her ex would wind up in court to make adjustments to the child support. She was constantly fighting with her kids. One fight had Judy wrestling on the floor with her daughter. There were 2 girls and one boy. I should have seen that this was a bad long-term situation for me, and I should have gotten out.

She wanted me to help her discipline the children—but her kids were here, while my own were 500 miles away in Buffalo at that time. I wasn't able to watch my daughters grow up and do things that would make me proud, or even discipline them when they needed it. As the wedding approached, I became more depressed and paranoid. I remember always thinking the Feds were after me. When I signed the Ketubah, a contract in Jewish marriages that ensures the groom will take care of the bride even if they divorce, I was really not all there. Even on our honeymoon, I thought the Feds were in the hotel with us. I remember standing on a balcony overlooking the pool and the lobby when I had this feeling. That feeling, that thought I had, tells me just how very sick I was.

I soon realized that I made a similar mistake with Judy that I had made with my first wife. When it was good between us, it was very good. When it was bad, the situation was not easy to live with.

She also resented any help I would give to my daughters, such as when I leased a car for Abigail. Judy thought I was using resources that should have gone to *her* kids, since we were married.

I reached rock bottom. Even during the day I felt dark, and I didn't want to share my feelings with anyone. Depression doesn't get any worse than suicide, and I wanted to end my life. I had to decide how to do it. Two weeks after we arrived home from the honeymoon, I got into my car and was planning to drive into a tree or telephone pole. I figured I would have to drive my car at about 65 miles per hour. I drove past tree after tree and just couldn't do it.

I also thought about jumping in front of a train and spent hours at a train station. I would stand at the edge of the platform. One train after another would speed by and I would just stand there and not have the guts to jump. Like driving into a pole, that was too difficult for me to follow through with, and I ended up taking a bottle of sleeping pills.

However, my reason for wanting to commit suicide had nothing to do with my marriage. If I wanted out of my marriage, there were less drastic ways. It was the paranoia that scared me the most. My mind went wild, thinking that I was constantly being watched by the Feds.

I went into our small downstairs bathroom and forced myself to swallow the pills. They knocked me out; my stepdaughter found me asleep the next morning with vomit coming out of my mouth and called 911, and I woke up in St. Charles Hospital. My head was foggy—a familiar feeling—and I felt disoriented. But there was a silver lining. This hospital stay is when I met Dr. Robert Castrol, who still is treating me today. At that time, he put me on a combination of Lithium, a mood stabilizing medicine; Zyprexa, an antipsychotic medicine that balances the levels of serotonin and dopamine in the brain; and Lamotrigine, an anti-seizure drug. He later added an anti-depressant called Alexapro to the mix (once again it was my sister who pushed for that) One more medication was added about four years ago called Atomoxetine also called Strattera commonly used for people with ADHD. It improved my concentration. This one was offered by my GP Dr. Polofsky. Dr. Castrol also prescribed my second series of shock treatments.

But while my head was clear, I was now confronted with explaining why I had tried to end my life within two weeks of my honeymoon. Oddly, I don't remember Judy's questioning my actions at that moment. She did grill me about it later, though, in a fit of rage.

My brother Ronnie committed suicide in 1997. He had an ear condition called hyperacusis which causes painful reactions to sound. It started as tinnitus when he played the drums in our band when we were teenagers. He had all the signs of someone who would commit suicide; it was obvious to all of us. He even practiced making a noose. Ronnie had to leave his job because of his hyperacusis and planted himself in his house. He wouldn't go out. We had to bring him food every day. We wanted him to get help and felt he might need medication, but he believed that meds would make his condition worse. He even belonged to the Hemlock Society, a right-to-die and assisted suicide advocacy organization, and my father helped him make out his Will. We finally forced Ronnie to go to a hospital. Our plan was to get him there just for the night, then take him to another hospital the next day.

It was the last place he wanted to be. They did a 10-minute intake, removed his watch but did not take his shoes and failed to put him on a suicide watch. In the morning, they found Ronnie dead in the shower, hung by his shoelaces. The hospital, and specifically his doctor, were negligent. We sued the doctor, but more importantly, we persuaded the State of New York to amend their protocol when dealing with a suicidal patient. There should always be a one-to-one watch.

My father passed away in 2005. My parents didn't always have an especially close relationship as I was growing up, but towards the end I saw them holding hands a number of times. That was touching to me.

My marriage to Judy was still very contentious. I walked on eggshells around her—I was always fearful of her outbursts. She was so mean-spirited. Our fights were very stressful and she was angry when I did anything for my children. This issue was the beginning of the end of our marriage.

It was hurtful to me that I couldn't be near my kids. I never had a chance to discover them as they grew up. Judy's kids were in school activities—the older girl was in chorus; the other daughter danced, and the boy, was in a band—and I would go to their concerts, really sad because my own kids weren't there.

I developed a bad habit: on weekends, I would stay in bed until around noon or later. This continued for a few years and would bother Judy greatly. I was just so unhappy living with her, I didn't want to face the day.

Jealousy was another strong emotion of Judy's, and her mood would swing often. I found this so difficult to deal with. We battled constantly. We tried marriage counseling, but it did no good. At that point, she started throwing my clothes outside, classic behavior that shows how someone despises you.

Finally, I simply left one night in 2003. Two days later, Judy committed suicide by taking pills. That made three people in my life who had committed suicide; if we counted my failed attempt, it would make four. I was conflicted about my feelings regarding Judy's death. Yes I was sad of course. I also felt a sense of relief. That was also sad. I was finally free of her and her children. The older boy moved in with his father. The girls already had places of their own.

Within 30 days of Judy's death, I moved into an apartment in Forest Hills. It was a great place; I could see Manhattan from my window. I was alone for the first time in a while and was moving on with my life very quickly. I joined Bally's Health Club and worked out three or four times a week. I already knew that physical exercise is very important for good mental health and builds brain cells. I also took private dance lessons for a year, though when the year was over, I still could not dance—I knew most of the steps but I could not feel the rhythm.

But I was still depressed. In 2007, I was having some problems at work. My boss called me on the phone on more than one occasion to suggest that I look for a new job. Once we met for dinner and he told me in person—he made it clear to me that he wanted me out, which caused me a great deal of stress. My depression deepened and of course the paranoia took hold again. I took enough pills to overdose.

My mom and Jackie saved my life. They had tried to call me—they normally called me at night—and when I didn't answer, they were alarmed and called the police. I was put in an ambulance and rushed to a hospital in Queens. Jackie brought Abigail and Amanda to visit me the next day—I wonder what that must feel like, to know your father tried to take his own life, not once but twice? It must have been hard for them to see me under those circumstances.

I was transferred to a hospital in Smithtown, in East Long Island, where Dr. Castrol practiced. I trusted him and wanted to be in his care.

I'm so happy I didn't take my life. From there, real healing began. I didn't know then what I know now, and I can honestly say, I am happier now than I've ever been before.

My mother died a natural death, from Parkinson's disease. Jackie and I had moved back into her home to care for her; we didn't send her to a nursing home or assisted living because we felt we could give her better care at home.. We worked hard to keep her alive, comfortable and relatively happy. Those years with mom were very special to me. I got to know her in a way I never had before. I truly adored her!

PART 3:

STILL THE SAME PERSON, BUT WITH A LOT LESS BAGGAGE

My recovery didn't materialize overnight, or even over a year's time, and it didn't happen in a straight line. In fact, it's still evolving. I have a wonderful network of supporters, and I'm able to observe and measure my progress as the months and years go by.

My recovery from depression encompasses five separate areas of my life, all complementing each other and interconnected in achieving my newfound health. I've listed them here, not necessarily in order of their importance:

- My work in a profession in which I can help people, and my ongoing determination to continue developing my skills and advance in that type of career;
- Enhance relationships with the people in my life;
- Exercise, exercise, exercise;
- Keep working on my awareness of my surroundings and appreciation of where I am, what I can accomplish and the kind of future I can create;
- The right medications and continued therapy-including my own mental exercises if I sense a change is coming.

Those are the five pillars that keep me elevated and strong. Each is essential to my recovery and rates some elaborating:

1. WORKING IN A HELPING PROFESSION AND DOING VOLUNTEER WORK

When Rev. Jefferson and his wife invited me to attend their Pentecostal church, and I stepped up to the podium and spoke to his congregation, I realized for the first time how healthy it felt to be helping people—and that's what I was doing, by sharing my story with Rev. Jefferson's parishioners. I truly believe that hearing about my challenges and recovery gave insights to those good folks about resolving difficulties in their own lives, especially if they were coping with a mental or emotional disorder, either theirs or a loved one's.

I've been back to his church a few times since then, and I will continue to attend whenever I can. My daughter Abigail has also attended with me, along with my grandson, Christian. I've told the pastor how much his invitation to speak has helped me, both in that moment and in the long run. I think that when someone does something that benefits you, it's always a good idea to let them know.

Working at a major pharmacy chain, and helping customers reach satisfaction in different areas, is something that enhances my mental and physical health almost every day. It picks me up, keeps my head on straight and is useful in handling negative behaviors.

Sometimes, helping customers is just a tiny thing—a smile, eye contact, or a friendly, kind remark about someone's haircut, for example. It helps me connect with them, makes both of us feel better, and if they're in the store with children I always make sure to give them a compliment about their kids if they deserve it.

This isn't the first outlet I've worked in. I was with another store in Amityville for about eight years and it closed, and all of us were relocated to our newest Amityville location. It can be a challenge; this store is the third-busiest store in the network. The people I work with are amazingly supportive of each other. We all like each other, actually. My attitude, working here, is more positive than I could ever have imagined on a job. I especially respect my boss. He never hesitates to get down in the trenches with us and do some of the grunt work, and he likes me. He is the kind of boss for whom you want to do a good job. He doesn't give out a lot of orders because we all know what we have to do, and he trusts that we will do our jobs. We work as a team.

I spend a good amount of time behind the cash register, and in that spot above all it's important to leave people with a smile. First impressions matter, as they say, but so do last impressions, and as customers are walking out the door, I want them to remember their visit as a positive part of their day. When people come to a pharmacy, they're either feeling good or they are there because they're not well and need something from the store or pharmacy. I can tell within five seconds if a customer is mean (or feeling mean that day), or if they're kind, just by the look on their face. They're either smiling or tight-lipped. A smile from me makes them feel better and lifts me up, too. I always remember to look them straight in the eye. Most shoppers feel that retail workers don't care about them, and I think it helps the world a little bit if I can change their thinking in some small way.

Being a happier person is a choice (if you are putting the five areas or pillars into practice), and helping people makes that choice easier. I'm 71 years old now, and there's something to be said for doing what makes you happy. One day, a co-worker mentioned to someone else that she was feeling depressed and had thoughts of hurting herself. I mentioned to her that I had tried to commit suicide and invited her to talk with me anytime. She's fine now, and it was a breakthrough for me to mention my suicide attempts to anyone outside the family.

I have worked at the pharmacy for almost 10 years now. Seven or eight years ago, Dr. Castrol, my psychiatrist, told me I was "in remission" from depression, and I think it had a lot to do with my workplace. I believe the job provided a "bridge" for me in my work life, between depression and wellness. It has been a great place to spend these years.

Now I'm kicking it up a notch with my ambition to work in a helping profession. In the spring of 2021, I had a conversation with a friend, a social worker named Karena. I told her I wanted to work in a helping profession, and she told me I should contact an organization called HALI (Hands Across Long Island). I called HALI's offices, and they suggested I look at the website of the Academy of Peer Services. It was while I was reading that website that I learned of a designation called a "Peer Specialist."

A Peer Specialist is a person who provides help and support to someone who is mentally challenged or dealing with an addiction, but earning that title is no simple matter. You can't just show up at a halfway house and start assisting residents.

The first step of the process involves rigorous training, a series of 13 core courses on subjects such as compliance and communicating with potential clients. Each of the classes involved three to four hours of work. All done on-line. Then you have to submit your application, including three references. Coming up with three solid references was a bit of a challenge; they couldn't be just anyone who knew me well, or even one who knew I was a responsible person. I wasn't allowed to use my doctors and was grateful that three professionals wrote letters recommending me for the program. The other requirement is that we were to have our own lived experience with mental health.

Finally, after training that spanned about six months, and my application was accepted, I had earned the title of "Provisional Peer" and was qualified to apply for a position with HALI. However, the training doesn't exactly end there; every two years I would have to be re-certified by taking and passing 15 credits of elective courses.

Some three weeks later, I called HALI. Instead of asking for a job, I told the person that I had completed the core 13 courses and was calling to learn how I might further my career. I was then put in touch with a man named Sal, who knows nearly everything about navigating HALI. He introduced me to his colleague Emily, who is in charge of the internship program there. I also learned there is a training class every Monday from 9:30 a.m. to 2:30 p.m.

And that's how I made my way into HALI's internship program. We had an orientation meeting, where I was able to meet the other interns, all of whom seemed to be nice, friendly people—which shouldn't be a surprise, since they, too, were looking to embark on careers in a helping profession.

In my first group session with the other interns, we talked about smoking and its harmful effects. There were six in the group, all of us trying to find a direction in this new-to-us field of helping others. I enjoyed the group meetings; they gave me a chance to talk about the good things happening to me and the problems I was overcoming, slowly but surely. Little did I know that I would form friendships in this group, Lydia and Kimberly . Both are younger than me. Lydia is a very smart woman who expresses herself extremely well. She has a huge heart. Lydia also is a great party planner with a real talent for bringing people together. Kim is a kind soul who remembers everyone. She likes to make gifts for people she cares about. She has made me a few.

During my internship, I was assigned to a group home. This was a residential program, where people lived who had issues that prevented them from living on their own at that moment. The particular home where I was assigned provided housing for 10 individuals. It was very clean and well organized. I meet with the residents Tuesday nights 5:00 p.m. to 9:00 p.m. and Friday mornings from 8:00 a.m. to 1:00 p.m.

During my first day, I spent some time reading Intake reports and reviews, getting to know the residents a bit through their paperwork. I learned very quickly that these folks have some serious issues and were coping with a lot in their lives. Yet, I felt strong empathy with them, because as I read through their reports, I was reminded of some of the things I had endured in my own life. Some of them were not so fortunate as I was. They didn't have my wonderful support system, and I pledged to be as supportive of these people as I could possibly be.

That same day, I visited another group home that housed four individuals who didn't need quite as much care as those in my group, and were somewhat more independent.

On my second day, I had fun playing Scrabble with my colleague and one of the residents. I was glad that I finally had the chance to get to know one of the residents.

At that time, I was reading a book by author Stephen King about how to write a book. I mentioned it to a resident, who is writing a book and he said that Stephen King was his favorite writer. When I left the CR (community residence, as the group homes are called) that afternoon, I went to Barnes & Noble and bought the book for him.

I gave him the book. He was so appreciative! He said it made him very happy, and I could tell that was true; he wasn't accustomed to having someone care about him as an individual with interests and skills of his own. And I couldn't have been happier, too. I want to make connections with all the residents. I want to make a difference in their lives.

I had a nice talk with another resident. She explained that she suffered from cerebral palsy and would be having surgery soon. We talked about her diamond painting, which was beautiful but she told me the tool she uses was not working. I offered to buy her another one, and I did—a tiny gesture that I know made a huge difference in her well-being right then. The diamond painting is done by placing tiny pieces of colored plastic onto a paper form which is a pretty design of some kind.

There was another resident who said little, so I engaged him in a game of Monopoly. He really enjoyed the game and talking with me.

One thing I have learned at the group home is that people like to talk about themselves. I suppose that's true of most people, but these were individuals who *needed* to talk about their lives and feelings. One resident was actually closed in, and I mean that literally and figuratively—he would stay in his room most of the day, and when he came out of his room, he barely spoke at all. People tended to avoid him because of his apparent preference for total solitude. One day, I asked John if he had any hobbies. He said he was a sculptor—and I have to say, a light went on in his head. It was as if no one had asked him about himself or his talents before. It turned out, John worked with wood, glass, copper and other metals, and he had his own website that showcased his sculptures. He took out his phone and showed me his art, and I showed him some of my father's art.

One thing to which he did pay attention was self-care. He was conscientious about getting a certain amount of exercise every day; he used a gym and even though he spent so much time in his room, he didn't enjoy sitting around, wasting time and smoking cigarettes, the way some residents did. I kind of liked him. I think we bonded. He was a good cooking partner.

Another woman at the home didn't know anything about cooking. In fact, there were no group dinners at the home; for the most part, residents bought their own food and stored it in cabinets, and they ate when and what they wanted. There was no cohesiveness. So I designated Tuesday nights "cook dinner night." We planned the menu on Friday and the staff had bought the food by the time I came in on Tuesday. We came together and made a different meal each week; pizza, stuffed pasta shells, chili, beef stew—whatever the residents had decided to put on the menu. Each person who participated had a job to do in preparing the meal, and we made a great team. The residents really enjoyed these "community" diners. This is a small example of how I knew I belonged in a helping profession, and could make a difference in people's lives: I was able to come up with ideas that made the residents' lives more enjoyable. I could help them grow into their best selves.

My work at the group home is interesting because it is the first job I've ever worked where I can truly be myself. In some other positions, I was required to wear a "mask." I have gone from helping municipalities raise money in the bond market to making dinner with residents of a group home, and this is where I do not need to wear a mask or hide anything about myself. (I also feel that freedom at the pharmacy.

When I say I can truly be myself at the group home, I compare it to floating on a raft with no noise and nobody around me. I am into myself and just enjoying my thoughts and thinking about the good people in this home. Experiencing that peace with myself is a feeling I have waited for a long time.

I'm at a place where I am continually thinking about my future. I finally feel as if I *have* a future.

I volunteer for a non-profit whose mission is to support people who have less than we do or are suffering from a terminal illness. During the summer, we offer a 5-day camp on a farm. This is primarily for kids with a terminal illness or who have had a major life disruption. There are games, arts and crafts, theater, a butterfly ceremony, a water slide, and a shaving cream fight. At Thanksgiving we distribute meals to needy families around Long Island. At Christmas we distribute gifts to more than 600 families. We had approximately 20 tour buses loaded with gifts and 8-10 volunteers on each bus. At each home we stopped at, we sang Christmas Carols and gave out the gifts.

The other non-profit is a service organization that raises money for various things such as food pantries, college scholarships for high school seniors, guide dog program and other charitable giving.

2. ENHANCING THE RELATIONSHIPS WITH THE IMPORTANT PEOPLE IN MY LIFE.

Jackie is a teacher in Brooklyn, New York and a smart woman—brilliant, in fact. She can hold a conversation on almost any topic; she remembers details of events and situations going back decades. I enjoy her company. She was the first to urge me to exercise. Jackie knew the benefits of exercise for good mental health and advocated for it, prodding me until I incorporated it into my daily routine. Along with my Doctors, I give Jackie credit for helping to lift me out of my fog. As I'm writing this, my awareness of my relationship with others has grown. I think it might be *me* who is causing the change, it could be that writing this book is therapeutic and somehow equips me to get a better handle on my everyday challenges.

And perhaps there's a message in there for anyone who lives with a stressful situation. We should all try to find a practice that bolsters us in that way, whether it's journaling, sketching, knitting, or engaging with nature. I think we all need to do something that gets us *into* the issues of our lives so we can be thoughtful about finding a healthy solution.

My older daughter, Abigail, is a trained hair stylist and now works in sales for a food distribution company. Abigail is smart, sensitive and a good mother to my grandson, Christian. Abby is always respectful of other people's opinions. She's a spiritual person, spending a lot of time praying and learning about God. She even sends me morning prayers that she wants me to use; I'm glad to see she has something in her life that she feels strongly about.

Abigail also is concerned that our country is headed for an economic depression and we might not have enough food available. So, she has been stockpiling food in her house and sends some to us—bags of pancake mix, oatmeal, sacks of cat food from Costco, a case of pork and beans. I finally told her not to send any more; we don't need it and don't have enough room for it. But this, too, is a strong belief of hers, and it's good to see her act on something she believes in. I think it's healthy. She's showing her intelligence and spirit.

I have two granddaughters by Amanda, my younger daughter — Blair and Sloan. I am Jewish but my daughters were raised Catholic, so we celebrate both Hanukkah and Christmas. Amanda married a Jewish man, Jared, and she converted to Judaism, so for her, spiritual matters have come full circle!

Amanda is a direct person and she is also kind. Amanda is an overachiever, excelling in everything she sets out to do, so it's no surprise that she is a good mother and a good wife. She works in real estate and does very well in her field.

I would be remiss if I didn't also mention the four-legged "people" in my life.

Jackie and I have three cats—Zachary, Oliver and Jamie. They're good to have around. Having a pet can be therapeutic and can help to relieve stress. There was one special dog in our family. Suzy lived with my Uncle Louie, who reached the age of 97. My aunt had died and Uncle Louie was living alone with Suzy; he lived in Amityville, not far from us, so I started going over to his house before work to take Suzy for a walk in the woods near their home. I could turn Suzy loose for a little while so she could run around the trees.

Eventually, Uncle Louie seemed to need more care, so I would make him breakfast, then return after work and walk Suzy again. My cousins really appreciated my helping out. When Uncle Louie's health was really failing, his biggest worry was that he didn't have anyone to leave Suzy with after he died. He was beside himself with worry over what would happen to Suzy.

I finally said that I would take Suzy, and Uncle Louie died very soon afterwards—it was as if he was waiting to resolve that one loose end before he could let go of his life. I found Uncle Louie gone in his bed, with Suzy lying beside him. It was a sweet, sad scene.

I took Suzy home with me; she was a good, happy dog. It wasn't long before she, too, died; she had a bad infection in her eye that never healed and we had to put her to sleep.

3. EXERCISE, EXERCISE, EXERCISE!

I started by running around the neighborhood. Soon I joined a gym, and once I had a gym membership it was easier to make exercise a regular part of my day. It was a time of frustration. I had gained some weight that I couldn't lose, so starting a strict routine (and sticking to it) was important.

I start early in the morning. That's the best time to work out, according to the National Institutes of Health, especially if you want to lose weight and keep it off—but the most important point is regular exercise, at whatever time of day suits you. I like to start early because it's a good way to start the day. It gives me positive energy—I like starting the day doing something worthwhile and optimistic for myself.

During my depression years, remember, I used to go to sleep to hide from people and the world, and there were periods when I would stay in bed for as long as I could. Now in my recovery, my purpose in going to sleep is to get up in the morning and start the day early. I am eager to face the world! I don't need a lot of sleep.

While at the gym my workout is simple and the same every day I am there. The first thing I do is about 20 minutes on the stair master (this is a great aerobic workout and also good for my legs). If you prefer something else you might try the treadmill, bicycle, or the elliptical machine. I then work my upper body. I use a different weight machine for each muscle. I work my biceps, triceps, shoulders, chest, and lats. I do 3 sets each of 8-12 reps for each muscle. My workout for my core is 3 sets each of 15-20 reps on a small incline. As time goes on I am looking to increase the number of reps. I then do 3 sets of leg lifts on an apparatus that allows me to hang from my arms. My core routine has changed over time. It is the most difficult part of my body to get good results. Diet is also important. I am at the gym 4-5 times a week. My workout takes about 1 hour and 15 minutes. If I can't go in the morning because of my work schedule I go in the evening.

We should all pay attention to our own bodies—I highly recommend using a trainer or fitness specialist of some sort, at the beginning when you're just learning how to use the machines safely and for maximum effectiveness. But listen to yourself as well, and make sure your trainer understands your needs and priorities. If you don't want to join a gym, you can get good information and videos online and from the library, and exercise at home. Even a fast walk around your neighborhood or exercising in your home to a "work out" video can make a big difference in your physical and mental wellness. Remember consistency is key.

4. AWARENESS OF MY SURROUNDING AND APPRECIATING MY LIFE.

This is sort of a collection of thoughts about what makes me feel good.

I now own and reside in the two-family home where I grew up. It's an Irish Tudor house style; I live on the first floor, and the upstairs apartment is rented to a nice couple. I have a deck and plenty of yard space, and I try to use it.

I drive a Honda CRV hybrid because both I am concerned about the environment, and I want to do our part in being responsible.

I do have some "things" that I cherish. If there's any possession that I treasure greatly, it would be a photograph of myself and my daughters when they were young. It was taken by my cousin Gary; it's well-composed and we all look happy. The girls are cute, and dressed nicely, and I keep the photo in my car (See the back cover).

Gary's father, my Uncle Abe, always wanted to take photos of prominent people. He took photos of the Duke and Duchess of Windsor, some of the Kennedys, and other luminaries. He worked for himself and he had a terrific talent for photography. Gary is talented, too.

I don't collect music, but I do like to hear it live. Live music feels therapeutic. Almost any kind of live music sounds good to me; I've heard the Philharmonic at Lincoln Center, Eric Clapton at Madison Square Garden, and I go to a jazz club in the city. I enjoy going to restaurants, too, often Japanese or Italian cuisine, or seafood restaurants. And I enjoy having dinner with a friend, cousin or other family.

5. TREATMENTS, THERAPY AND MEDICATIONS.

I have a team that watches over me. The team consists of my psychologist, my psychiatrist and my sister.

My sessions with my therapist, Dr. Michael Herships, are by phone, every Thursday afternoon at 4:30. I enjoy working with him; he has a way of making sense out of an awkward thought or issue I need to talk about. Somehow, my problems seem to fade when I discuss them with Dr. Herships; they seem much smaller. Also, we do have some fun during our sessions.

We talk about anything and everything going on in my life. There are one or two major issues that he cannot make disappear so easily, such as the need for approval and validation. He has provided me with enough thoughts, enough mental and emotional tools, to manage them. Most people are surprised to learn that the chemicals in your brain are affected by psychotherapy, but it's true. During therapy, the patient talks to a licensed, trained medical professional who helps the patient identify and work through the factors that might trigger their depression. That much is obvious; those sessions help the patient understand their behaviors, ideas, and emotions that contribute to his depressed state.

Eventually, with enough therapy, the patient is able to control those behaviors and ideas, and feel peace and pleasure again. Along the way, he will learn coping techniques and problem-solving skills—not only through talking with the therapist one-on-one, but also through group, couples and family therapy, if those avenues are relevant to the patient's life.

The most effective therapy or intervention, says the American Psychiatric Association, is cognitive behavior therapy (CBT), an approach that helps individuals change negative thoughts and behaviors. In fact, some 75 percent of patients treated with CBT benefit from it. We spent a fair amount of time working through my need for constant approval.

Now here's the technical explanation of how psychotherapy changes your brain chemicals—apologies for all the jargon, but this is really interesting:

Psychotherapy "produces long-term changes in behavior by producing changes in gene expression that alter the strength of synaptic connections and structural changes that alter the anatomical pattern of interconnections between nerve cells of the brain." (Those are the findings of a study published in the Indian Journal of Psychiatry in 2017.)

That's a mouthful, but in simpler terms, therapy *actually can change the brain's architecture and mechanisms and help to rebuild the broken parts.*

The real-life results of these brain-changes are fewer medical problems, fewer sick days, and a genuine increase in work satisfaction. CBT contributes to these outcomes by rewiring the brain. CBT "coaches" the brain chemicals, over time, to follow different pathways, thereby changing the patient's behavior in positive ways. I told you it was interesting stuff.

Dr. Robert Castrol, my psychiatrist, prescribes and monitors my medications. You might remember, I met Dr. Castrol after my first suicide attempt, and he arranged for me to be transferred to a different hospital so that he could treat me. He has given me the proper "cocktail" of meds that have stabilized me and given me hope that I can forever live a normal, healthy life. One of the medications was Lithium which I have been on for over 20 years. It started to harm my kidneys. Dr. Castrol was very reticent about replacing it. I finally convinced him to take me off and the thought was to put me on Depacote. We took me off the Lithium and did not give me the Depacote. We wanted to see how I would do without it. I have been doing great. This is an important milestone in my recovery. For me to rid myself of a medication I depended on for such a long time is a major accomplishment. We talk every four weeks. I believe he can tell how I am feeling just by talking to him.

Dr. Castrol always likes to talk about the "dating scene" and tells me stories about how people he knows have found their life partners. He's always pushing me to keep trying to find a woman!

Psychoanalysis certainly helps me. If my brain chemicals change, it relieves some stress that I'm feeling—and if I'm able to feel more relieved, I'm better at conquering situations that, in the past, caused me stress. Eventually, I can replace it with a positive thought. It goes back to my childhood that created those feelings of needing approval. Now that I am healthier, I am experiencing something new. I now know what it is to have a truly positive attitude at work, and even better, what it means to take a negative thought and replace it with a positive thought.

These are things I've never experienced in my entire life. Maybe I have taken a step closer to realizing a more complete happiness. I won't be completely there until I can control my negative feelings.

So the negative thinking is still lurking—but I am better! I recognize it and do a mental work-around and keep going. It's not automatic yet, but it's getting there.

The third member on this team is my sister, Jackie. She reads me like a book. She is on the lookout for any major shift in my mood. If that happens, she would push me to talk with one or both of my doctors. Jackie always has my back!

I would be remiss if I did not mention my GP Dr. Polofsky. He prescribed a medication called Atomoxatine or better known as Stretera. This is commonly used to treat people with ADHD. It helps keep me focused.

SOME CLOSING THOUGHTS:

I still feel a little anxiety sometimes. I worry about my longevity (I'm 71 years old at this writing), but then I see people at the Pharmacy who are younger than me and don't look well. I also see customers who are much older than me, and they look great. I'm healthy and free of disease. I also know it's not the number of years that matters most, it's the quality of one's life that's really important. I need to relax and let that sink in.

I'm doing many positive, healing things for myself—the exercise, counseling, meds, self-love.

I'm very fortunate, because of the way I was found when my mom and my sister called the police to rescue me when I didn't call that night, that I was saved from ending my life. I'm especially blessed that I no longer have to wear a mask of any kind.

My healing has taken what feels like a lifetime. The most important messages of this book, and the primary reason why I wanted to write it: let's erase the stigma our society has attached to mental illness and that you or no one else did anything that caused the illness. Also very importantly I show how to get well.

Depression, bipolar disorder and other mental conditions are not labels, and they don't make you less than anyone else. You can go forward and make a life that's as normal as everyone else's—work, exercise, go to concerts, travel, cook, have a family, laugh with friends. Laugh and laugh. Find good support— you've got this!

EPILOGUE:

A BRIGHT NEW BEGINNING

I am thrilled to add a new chapter to this book, and to my life: I have achieved my goal of working in a helping profession! Beginning this new career is an important step in my longtime quest to earn my living by helping people. It's not an easy job, and I couldn't be happier.

My official title is Direct Service Professional. I started this job on June 15, 2023; my employer is a company that works with people who have various mental disorders. Most have been diagnosed with autism; a few might occasionally try to hurt themselves or even become violent. This is not a residential program; clients arrive by bus at about 9:00 a.m., most coming from the group homes where they live, and spend much of the day with us. Approximately 30 clients attend our program every day, ranging in age from their early 20s to mid-30s, and the ratio of clients to staff is excellent: 1 staff to 3 clients plus there are three managers that are there at all times during the day.

The job began with two weeks of training. We were taught to deal with all sorts of circumstances, from engaging and communicating with clients who do not talk, to defusing potentially dangerous situations. People with certain mental disorders have a tendency to act out, and we have to be ready to make sure the client, and everyone in the area is safe. The usual protocol is to subdue the client until he or she calms down. We use specific techniques to make that happen.

Our primary goal is to keep the clients busy and try to engage them in some activity, hopefully helping them improve their skills along the way. This happens on various levels, depending on the individual's skills. They might color or do word games or puzzles. One man, for instance, is learning to keep his workspace clean and put things away when he's not using them. Some clients work at computers; one practices his computer skills by copying ads from the computer onto his tablet. I'm working with another to learn addition—we can print "activity sheets" for whatever tasks clients perform on any given day—and this client understands the math problems but doesn't know how to write the numbers properly. So, I have to guide his hand and make sure he writes the numbers as he solves the problems. Some need a little direction and lots of encouragement while others may just need to be by themselves in their own world.

I look for the little things they do, the small rewards that come when I least expect them, that let me know a client understands. Here is an example: A client was working at a computer. I went over to him and asked him his name. He said something, but I could not understand what he was saying, so I asked him to repeat it. I still couldn't understand him. He had a tablet, so I asked him if he would type his name on his tablet. He did—his name is Christopher. I spoke his name, but he didn't respond. But then I said "Chris," and he gave me a thumbs-up—he wants to be called Chris, not Christopher. This is one of those things that are special and that keeps me going. Here is another example. I had set my keys down on a table next to a nice lady a client who does not talk at all. I had signed a form next to her and forgot about the keys and I walked away. I came back a minute or two later and there she was holding up my keys with a smile, I took the keys and I said, "Thank you," and she gave me a high sign—it was cute and just a small gesture, but it was communication. It was progress.

On some days, we take the clients on excursions, five or six at a time, with two staffers. We take them to the library, or the gym, or to a park. I like to get out for these excursions, and the clients enjoy them, too. The last time we went to a park for a couple of hours, we all ate lunch there, in the fresh air.

What I like most about the job is working with the clients—taking good care of them and seeing them respond to me. I love that interaction with them. Every day, something good happens that reminds me that my journey is worthwhile.

All of my co-workers are younger than me, but a handful have been there a while. They understand the clients' behaviors, their relationships, and they recognize their triggers. They're savvy about the job, and I learn from them. We are a great team, we have each other's back. The hardest part of working here is getting clients to focus on one thing at a time. I'm trying to teach one guy, for instance, how to do a better job of coloring. All he does is scribble, he doesn't try to color one section at a time, and I'd like to see him develop that skill.

I have a lot of respect for the management. They are not afraid to roll up their sleeves and get involved with the tough stuff

I came here from the pharmacy, a workplace where I respected the people and appreciated what I could accomplish there. However, it became routine—a little too steady and predictable. I was ready to stretch my legs, learn new skills and begin my career in a helping profession. And that might be the biggest difference between then and now: that was a job, and this is a *career*. It's an important distinction. I needed to start a career in which the days are a bit uncertain. I needed to know that I can feel comfortable—*not stressed*, at least not in a bad way—in work that is different every day. When I've helped a client produce a good outcome, that's when I'm happiest. That's when I feel the most comfortable. It's a challenge if I have to persuade them to sit down and try to learn something, but challenges are good. We always go back to learning and being productive together. Even a little smile is a big deal for some and that may be enough for one day.

And the rewards keep coming.

APPENDIX A:

EXPLAINING DEPRESSION AND BIPOLAR DISORDER IN CHILDREN

Readers might be surprised to learn that children can be diagnosed with depression—and, in fact, doctors now recognize it as early as age 3.

Depression is a relatively new diagnosis for kids. Psychiatrists and psychologists were observing their depressive behaviors and symptoms in the 1940s, but it wasn't until the 1970s that the illness was seen as a valid disorder that needed medical treatment.

The symptoms usually are easy to spot in children: they seem sad, hopeless, or irritable much of the time. Their "cranky" moods translate to not wanting to participate in activities they would normally enjoy.

Some of the same behaviors are seen in children with bipolar disorder, which is most often diagnosed in older children and teens, but can happen at any age: as with adults, youngsters with bipolar disorder can experience mood swings ranging from euphoria (often referred to as "mania") to lows of serious depression. In a manic phase, the child can be aggressive or hyperactive, irritable and exhibiting socially inappropriate behaviors. They may also show signs of insomnia, and experience what's known as an "ADHD meltdown"—a sudden outburst of frustration and anger. In some combinations, these symptoms can be similar to those of ADHD, so the child is sometimes misdiagnosed. About 20 percent of people with ADHD also have bipolar disorder.

In the lower phases the child might feel very low energy and other emotions similar to those felt with depression: sadness, hopelessness, guilt, self-doubt and pessimism. The child might also have difficulty concentrating or remembering things.

The causes of both depression and bipolar disorder are difficult to pinpoint. If parents display patterns of irritability or withdrawal, that can lead to a child's developing low self-esteem and predisposing him or her to depression later in life. Depression in kids also is associated with a family history of mood disorders and other psychiatric conditions. Bipolar disorder, too, is thought to be caused by a combination of physical, environmental and social factors, and is often inherited. In fact, genetics account for about 80 percent of the source of bipolar disorder, according to a research institute in Australia.

Diagnosing mental disorders in children is a process involving a physical exam, lab tests and a psychological evaluation. The most important thing is, if you know a child whose behavior has changed recently or seems odd, talk to a medical or mental health professional as a first step. With professional treatment, support and love from family and friends, kids and teens not only will get better faster, they will be more likely to avoid mental health problems in their future.

Sources: Mayo Clinic; Centers for Disease Control and Prevention

APPENDIX B:

HOW HELPING PEOPLE HELPS DEPRESSION

I've written about my quest to be of service to people for a living—to work full-time in a helping profession. Turns out, scientists say that goal makes sense for someone like me, a man with depression.

Performing acts of kindness boosts your own sense of well-being, say researchers for the Mental Health Foundation in the United Kingdom. Simply put, being an "actively kind" person makes you feel better about *yourself*. It also gives you a great opportunity to strengthen or grow your own support networks, and encourages you to be more active—which in turn increases your self-esteem.

Putting the needs of others before your own can make a big difference in your quality of life, according to Behavioral Health Systems, Inc., a U.S.-based organization that provides mental health services for its members. That sort of other-directed behavior can lower your stress level, improve your mood and generally increase your happiness, all of which promotes endorphins (hormones that block pain and give you a sense of well-being) in your brain through positive physiological change. In other words, *helping others actually alters your brain chemistry in a positive way!*

And that's not all you can transform; you can enhance your immune system by doing good deeds. Being a "giving person" actually makes you healthier!

The proof is in the studies—older people who frequently assist others, live longer than those who don't.

It's a proven fact: the more you help others, the more you help yourself!

APPENDIX C:

THE IMPORTANCE OF EXERCISE, ESPECIALLY CARDIO, IN HELPING TO FIGHT DEPRESSION.

It's a fact: Depression makes you feel physically crummy, and it's sometimes a downward spiral, according to the Harvard Medical School blog ("Harvard HealthBeat"). You get less sleep, which gives you less energy during the day, which gives you aches and pains, which lowers your motivation to exercise.

But studies show that exercise can be as effective as antidepressants. If you are severely depressed, exercise alone will not heal you—but it will help.

Exercise "starts a biological cascade of events that results in many health benefits," a Harvard study states, including protecting you against heart disease and diabetes, improving sleep patterns and lowering blood pressure. It also releases endorphins, our "feel-good chemicals" in our brains, so it boosts our mood, too.

For most people, the biggest value of exercise over time is that it triggers the release of proteins called neurotrophics or growth factors—our nerve cells grow and make new connections, bringing an improvement in brain activity and actually making us feel better.

The *hippocampus*—the part of our brain that helps regulate our mood—is smaller in depressed people than in the general population. But with exercise, the nerve cells in our hippocampus will grow, nerve cell connections improve, and little by little, depression is relieved.

If you are depressed and cannot make yourself exercise, the experts recommend moving *just a little*. Walk for five minutes—down your street, back and forth in your living room, wherever you are comfortable. Even exercising for those few minutes will elevate your mood *over time*. Doing it consistently, every day, is more important than adding more time. When you're ready to add more time to your daily workout, your body—and your mind—will let you know.

APPENDIX D:

DEPRESSION OR BIPOLAR DISORDER—WHICH IS IT?

I understand why the two illnesses are often confused—and if the doctors can't even pinpoint our illnesses, how can we?

So, I thought it would be helpful to readers if I would outline a few of the differences here. These notes are gathered from the National Institutes of Health website and other scholarly sources.

Depression and bipolar disorder are often confused because bipolar disorder can include depressive episodes. The essential difference is that depression is *unipolar*, meaning that there is no "up" period. Bipolar disorder, which is sometimes called "manic depression," on the other hand, includes symptoms of mania. It's characterized by extreme mood swings, and many people with bipolar disorder experience both manic and depressive episodes.

The symptoms are often triggered by a stressful situation. It can be a singular event, such as losing a job, but it can also be an ongoing situation. Depression can go on for as long as months, or even years and it can require medication or a hospital stay.

Manic symptoms include high energy, excitement, impulsive behavior, and agitation.

Depressive symptoms are the opposite: a lack of energy, feeling worthless, low self-esteem, and sometimes suicidal thoughts. Depression can run in families, but heredity is not the only factor. The ADA and Social Security Administration, by the way, consider bipolar a disability. Bipolar can develop at any age, often between the ages of 15 and 19, rarely after 40, most often in a person's 20s. It doesn't go away and requires a lifetime of treatment. But a person can develop skills to better manage both manic and depressive episodes.

Also, certain substances can trigger symptoms: alcohol, hallucinogens (LSD, PCP), antidepressants, heart medications, blood pressure medications, prescription pain relievers, and decongestants. These substances *cannot* cause bipolar, but can trigger symptoms in a person who has the disease.